Belly Fat

Summer Body Workouts:

Simon Roche

Finicky Inc.

New York

FREE Bonus: [https://healthresultswealth.wordpress.com/ **]**
Motivational Coffee

Hi, my name is Simon Roche, Founder of "Finicky.us" and also the author to many entrepreneurial and self-help books.

I have seen that I was different since I was a kid. When other kids wanted to play, I wanted to be productive and better myself. Not to say that I didn't play on my free time, I just didn't play longer than I needed. I always set my expectations out of my reach and I truly hope that my readers do the same. I have visited many companies during my career and I can say that I have learned more than if I were to have worked for a company.

As a thank you for considering my book, I will provide you with one of my many experiences while visiting a friend at Google. My friend who was previously the "Strategic Partner Lead" at Google has had many accomplish through his career and no longer works at

Google. We became friends in our marketing course and have still kept in contact.

He gave me a tip about the process of hiring people for my company. During the selection process, he weaves out many strong candidates. Why? Simply because they aren't smarter than me, the interviewer. He explains that if you want a good company, then you surround yourself with average brains that just want to get by. At Google, we don't want average, we want the smartest. Smart people hire smarter people and that's how Google is still on top of its industry. He stated, "I want to hire someone who is smarter than me, works better than me, and is more innovative than me. That way I will be happy when they take my position, as I move on to another chapter in my life"

Through my books, I will share many of my unique experiences and will provide you with mistakes that I have made myself as an entrepreneur.

Before you start reading this book, I will need you to keep a thought in mind.

"To be able to sacrifice what you are, for who you will become"

In other words, if you put aside your excuses, you will get the results you have always wanted. It's time to make a decision. You can choose to stay the way you are or you can decide to take steps towards change.

No one is stopping you from where you want to go, the only person that is stopping you is YOU. Remind yourself every day of who you want to be, and remember to make the right decisions towards your goal. One way to keep your goals set is by checking up on yourself at the end of each week. Set a goal for 2 pounds each week, and by the end of the month you will have cut 8 pounds. Keep your short-term goals small so that it is achievable, but keep your long-term goals big, so that there is no ceiling towards your success.

Losing Weight with (HIIT) High Intensity Interval Training

Throughout my fitness experience, the more I interviewed my clients it became apparent that so many people were aspiring for a specific yet very common look. But, what these clients really wanted was the positive physical change and confidence that came as a result of leading a healthy lifestyle.

In this book we are going to focus on high intensity interval training as a very effective weight loss tool among other benefits. My main mission is to help as many people as possible achieve their ideal body, happiness and unmatched confidence!

The fitness world is very dynamic and every day there is something new coming up that is deemed to be the best fat blaster. There are so many different things and products in the market that all promise to give the best results, available shortcuts and all the things you should do and those that you should avoid. In this book, I am hoping to dispel all the rumors, clear the confusion and focus more on your weight loss goals.

If you are stuck in a 45 minute daily exercise routine and are not really seeing any major changes in your weight loss efforts, then this is going to be a real eye opener. But first, let us look at the definition of HIIT workouts.

The What

"High-intensity interval training (HIIT), also called High-Intensity Intermittent Exercise (HIIE) or sprint interval training, is an enhanced form of interval training, an exercise strategy alternating periods of short intense anaerobic exercise with less-intense recovery periods. HIIT is a form of cardiovascular exercise. Usual HIIT sessions may vary from 9–20 minutes. These short, intense workouts provide improved athletic capacity and condition, improved glucose metabolism and improved fat burning"

HIIT is one of the best proven ways to burn fat. It's basically cardio on steroids, so to say, as it combines intervals of very intense exercises like sprinting with intervals of complete rest or low intensity exercises such as jogging or walking. HIIT is the complete opposite of LISS (Low Intensity Steady State) that most people do for periods lasting between 30-60 minutes.

The HIIT technique was developed years ago by track coaches to increase runners' speed and endurance for better athletic performance. It was first referred to as **Fatlek** – coined from two Swedish words, **fart** (speed) and **lek** (play). This is probably one of the main reasons why HIIT is very strongly associated with athletic performance rather than being a training technique for someone looking to burn fat and get toned.

The first rule of HIIT is '**No pain no gain**'. This is because this form of exercise is based on sheer intensity and hard work. You feel every muscle and fiber in your body respond to the grueling exercises and you can be 100 hundred percent sure that if you stay true and consistent, you are going to achieve your ideal body in a matter of weeks!

The Who

"I have never done any intense workouts in my life, the most I have done is walk for 40 minutes. At first I lost 5 pounds just from walking but of late I seem to have stagnated. I hear that HIIT really works but it is mostly use by well-seasoned athletes and workout bunnies. Can I still do HIIT and see the pounds shift?"

In a nutshell – YES!

HIIT is a very dynamic exercise technique and can be performed by virtually everyone. It doesn't matter if you are a newbie and can only manage one or two sessions in a week or a pro athlete who can do HIIT session 5 days in week. Whether you are looking to gain muscle or shed body fat, HIIT will help you meet your goals. Period!

Most body builders usually shy away from cardio as it stimulates slow twitch muscle fibers that build endurance. With time, your muscles can become smaller and weaker or you can eventually reach a plateau where no matter how much you train you won't be gaining muscle.

To better understand this, compare marathon runners with sprint runners. Marathoners are smaller and far less muscular and this can be directly attributed to the low impact steady state routine that they do on a regular basis. On the other hand, sprinters are muscular, compact and have a denser appearance. This is because they regularly train their fast twitch muscle fibers that are built for speed. The reason why marathoners look so thin is because their bodies mostly comprise of slow twitch muscle fibers that take less time for nutrients to travel within the fibers and thus speed up the rate at which the nutrients are burned for fuel to sustain the long runs.

To understand this better, think of it this way; by arguing that LISS is best for maintaining muscle mass is like saying that performing 5-pound dumbbell curls for half an hour will build you more muscle compared to performing 40-pound dumbbell curls for 4 sets for 10 reps each with short intervals of rest of 30seconds in between sets. Who do you think will build more muscle, the one lifting heavy weight or the one lifting 5-pound weights?

A study carried out in New Zealand showed that HIIT triggered the production of more testosterone compared to LISS and since testosterone plays a very important role in muscle development, it means that HIIT can actually boost muscle growth and strength.

What about losing weight?

 Well, if shedding fat is your main goal or torching the love-handles around your mid-section so you can rock a summer bikini – you are in the right place. HIIT is definitely what you need! One of the reasons why HIIT is a great hit for those interested in losing weight is its 'after burn' ability. This training technique produces EPOC (Excess Post Exercise Oxygen Consumption).

In simple terms, what this means is that your body experiences an increased rate of oxygen intake after an intense workout that is basically intended to expunge your body's 'oxygen debt'. An important thing to note is that you have to perform HIIT exercises properly for o to enjoy its benefits. Some people for instance assume that interval cardio – alternating intensity and speed intervals, qualify as HIIT, when actually that's not the case.

Interval cardio pushes you to (65-85) % of your maximum heart rate. HIIT however should push you to a minimum of 85% which is actually training until your muscles feel like they are burning!

The How...

 One of the most important things about HIIT exercises is to understand how to use them properly to achieve your goals. As we saw previously, HIIT training is great for high calorie burn which translates to fat loss. However, too much of it can lead to stagnation or chronic fatigue (overtraining) and that is why it is important to know exactly how to perform HIIT routines.

For beginners...

Newbies are the most susceptible to injury and overtraining and here is the reason:

1. When starting out, most people are very excited to go after their dream body that they bite off more they can chew without even knowing it. When beginning a new fitness regimen the motivation and drive kicks in super hard and every person wants results fast! And so the natural instinct is to go really hard and fast from the get-go.
    Unfortunately, your body is yet to be ready for intense workouts and not just because you lack the strength or endurance but also from the

lack of central nervous system development and exercise technique needed to execute HIIT correctly.

The truth is, you need to learn—actually, earn—your way into super intense body workouts. The truth is, it takes time, patience and practice to develop the skills and physiology that will enable you to HIIT like a pro!

2. When starting out many Newbies have some level of difficulty in knowing how to assess and set resting periods between intense workouts. During intense exercises, your body is stressed and your tissues are broken down and it is therefore very important to plan rest and recovery time well in order to increase your fitness level.

So many times however, either due to over-ambition or poor coaching, most of us don't allow enough resting periods which can lead to overtraining and injury.

For beginners, I find that the best HIIT exercise to start on is the bike; because it is one directional and very easy on the joints compared to sprinting that can give you some unpleasant injuries such as runner's knee. Starting on a bike leaves enough room for error, allowing you to slowly ease yourself into HIIT training.

Intermediate and pro levels

Your biggest concern should be whether adding HIIT training to your profile of workouts is going to help you achieve your goals. Considering you have been working out for quite some time now, your body is going to be in a position to make the necessary adaptations to handle the added stress from high intensity workouts.

It is also very important to clearly define your goals;

❖ I want to put on muscle

You should limit HIIT workouts to two sessions in a week

❖ I want to shed body fat and become lean

You can perform HIIT for 3-4 times in a week depending on your body's ability to recover well.

❖ I want to build endurance for sprinting...

If your goal is to increase your running time per mile or if you want to increase you capability of going for rounds in say boxing, HIIT can be done as often as possible for as long as you leave out enough recovery time.

❖ **I want to build endurance for long distance running**

If you are looking to go for a triathlon or a marathon, HIIT will not do much to help you as it works on building your fast twitch muscle fibers but, for long distance running, you need slow twitch muscle fibers to be well developed.

❖ **I want to build strength**

You should only perform HIIT once a week, ensuring you recover fully before going back to your lifting schedule.

Blast more fat

We have established that you burn a lot of calories during a HIIT workout, but that's not all. Your body goes though intense exertion that launches the repair cycle. You therefore burn more calories and fat for the 24 hours after your intense workout, more than say after a LISS workout.

A healthy heart

Not many of us can attest to having reached the anaerobic zone – the place where you push yourself hard to the point you literally can't breathe and you feel like your heart wants to jump out of your chest. Extreme HIIT produces amazing results such as making your heart stronger by making your blood vessels more elastic and better able to expand.

A recent study on HIIT found that the subject could cycle two times longer than they could before whilst cycling at the same pace.

You don't need any equipment

Jumping rope, cycling, running and even rowing are great for HIIT and what's even better is that you don't need any equipment. Fast feet, high knees, jumping lunges or any other plyometric exercise like burpees work on getting your heart rate up very fast.

Lose fat and NOT muscle

If you have been on a diet before, you know that it's very hard not to lose muscle as you lose fat. Studies have shown that LISS seemingly encourages muscle loss as well. However, weight training and HIIT routines ensure most of the weight loss comes from depleted fat stores and that muscle mass is preserved.

Boost your metabolism

Apart from preventing muscle mass, HIIT boosts the production of the human growth hormone (HGH) during the 24 hours after your HIIT routine. HGH not only increases calorie burn but it also helps you stay younger y slowing down the aging process both inside and outside.

You can do it anywhere

All you need to do is to move at your maximum effort for a short amount of time followed by a rest period and repeat the process. This is all you need to do for a successful HIIT session so, whether you are on a boat, a bicycle or on your own two feet, get to action and get the most out of your training.

Always up for a challenge

Are you tired of doing easy exercises that you can even read a magazine or work on your computer while doing? Well, HIIT is all you need. Because of how short the actual workout session is, you will be working extremely hard all the time. You will feel the burn in your muscles and you may end up sucking wind, but one thing is for sure, you are going to shed weight fast and you definitely won't be bored when doing so.

Curb your appetite

You may have wrongly assumed that engaging in intense exercise makes you super hungry. However, a study by the University of Western Australia showed that ghrelin, the hormone responsible for stimulating hunger was suppressed in the subjects who were performing HIIT, and thus decreasing their appetite significantly reducing your appetite for a period after your training session.

Fast and furious

Have you been shying away from getting fit because you simply don't have time to spare? Well, HIIT is an amazing way of squeezing in a great workout in the shortest amount of time. The fact is that you can achieve maximum results in a session that is as short as 10 minutes. You should note that due to the extreme intensity of the HIIT routine, you get all the benefits of a strenuous gym session in a matter of minutes. As the name suggests, HIIT is fast and furious.

Many of us have tired as much as 5 different fitness regimes in the bid to lose weight and achieve our dream body. But many are the times we throw in the towel 1, 2, 3 or 4 week into the regimen, especial if it is steady state cardio. There are so many reasons why this happens and it's not because you are a failure or do not have enough willpower.

Steady state cardio can become easily monotonous especially if you do the same routine day in day out without a change in scenery. Another thing with steady state cardio is that you may only note significant weight loss changes for a certain period of time and slowly as your body adjusts and gets used to your exercise regimen, reach a plateau where no matter how much you run, bike or swim, you don't note any changes to be excited about.

This is where tabata comes in. would you believe you can achieve your weight loss goals by working out for just 4 minutes? Sound too good to be true? Well, let us delve deeper into tabata training and see how this unique HIIT routine is going to change your life!

Tabata training owes its existence to Dr. Izumi Tabata and a small team of researchers in Tokyo in the National Institute of Fitness and Sports. They used two groups of athletes where one trained at a steady, moderate level while the other group trained at a very high intensity level.

The first group that trained at a moderate level had 5 training sessions in a week for a total of 6 weeks and each session lasted for one full hour. On the other hand, the second group had 4 training sessions in a week for a total of 6 weeks and each session lasted for 4 minutes and 20 seconds, with 10 seconds of rest after each set.

Results

Group one that operated on a moderate state workout had increased their overall cardiovascular system but had little or no results for the muscular (anaerobic system).

Group two that was on a high intensity training schedule showed a greater increase in their cardiovascular system as well as their anaerobic system which they had increased by 28%.

Their study concluded that HIIT has a greater impact on both aerobic and anaerobic systems.

TABATA

Four minutes of working out may not seem to be adequate for any visible physical change but I can assure you that these four minutes are going to be the longest four minutes of your life! Seeing stars, feeling your heart burn within your chest cavity, nausea, sucking wind... this is exactly how you now that you are doing your tabata right! At first you might be wondering why the hell would you want to intentionally do this to your body, but what you stand to gain from this extreme four-minute workout outweighs the shirt-lived discomfort.

Those who have been on tabata rightfully dub it 'the four minute miracle'

The 3 most important rules of tabata are:

1) Although you can do tabata intervals with virtually all exercise routines, it is important to start with a routine that you are familiar and comfortable with. If you have been doing steady state running, you should try sprinting; if you have been jumping rope, stick to that but now follow the tabata sequence, if you have been doing weights, incorporate a tabata

interval...basically, start with the known before venturing to the unknown so you can ease your body gently into this routine.

2) An accurate timer is of utmost importance when it comes to tabata. No matter how good you are at estimating time, you cannot accurately estimate 10 second and 20 second intervals when your brain is all worked up and fuzzy. You will need to focus all your energies to the exercise at hand and not have to keep asking yourself whether the 20 seconds have elapsed.

3) Get a good and motivational mantra to recite in time with your footfalls for the 20 seconds burst. This may sound a bit silly but you need something else to focus on and not the excruciating pain rocking your body. This mantra will also help you feel like thee 20 seconds don't last long.

The basic structure of the tabata workout is:

- Workout really hard for 20 seconds straight
- Take 10 second rest
- Do eight complete rounds

As we have established, you don't have to labor for hours on your elliptical or treadmill to burn off the excess fat. All you need is four minutes for four to five times a week. The amazing thing about tabata is that it is not just confined to running, jumping rope or solely aerobic exercises, you can incorporate numerous exercises to get the most out of your workouts. You can choose to train wit just your bodyweight or you can kick it up a notch by adding duels, barbells and kettle bells.

The trick is knowing how to do it, if for example you want to incorporate tabata into your weight training routine, just select four barbell exercise that you can comfortably transition between and start by performing the first set by doing the maximum possible reps you can within a span of 20 seconds, take a rest for 10 seconds then take on the next exercise for the next 20 seconds, again as may reps as possible, rest for 10 seconds and repeat this training process or the remaining exercises all for a total of 4 minutes.

Take caution with tabata!

Not the best exercise for beginners

Owing to the fact that tabata is very intense, it is best for advanced and well-seasoned trainers who have mastered the art of high intensity exercises. How tabata work is that the intensity gradually accumulates reaching its peak near the end. This can easily become overwhelming and extremely challenging if you are not used to high intensity interval training and you may find yourself throwing in the towel way too soon.

The key is to gradually increase the intensity of your training, putting in enough recovery periods in between the exercises. Start with simple exercises such as running, jumping rope, swimming and rowing then progress to squats, pushups when you are more comfortably. Then with time you can now incorporate tabata into your regimen.

Risk of injury

Tabata involves going all out during the high intensity bursts and so there is always risk of injury. However, you can minimize this risk by increasing your fitness levels to ensure your body can handle the maximum exertions from such exercises. Another thing you should do before performing tabata is to do a complete warm up to ensure your body is ready to take on the grueling exercise session.

Risk of monotony

Fur minutes may not seem like much time for something to get monotonous but, performing the same type of exercise day in day but, even with rest periods can cause your motivation and form to suffer. Your muscles will know what to expect and won't work as hard as they should. Prepare different sets of exercises that you can switch p so you are always looking forward to the new and challenging experience.

Mental strength

When pushing yourself to the limit with tabata, the four minutes may seem like a lifetime. It may be quite intense and the urge to give it all up will be so strong but always carry a mental image of how you are going to look like if you persist and keep going like a champ!

Nutrition watch

Just because you are working out your body to a T does not mean you have the license to eat whatever you want. For fastest weight loss results, the general rule is that nutrition works 80 % while exercise works the remaining 20%.

When doing HIIT exercises such as tabata, you need to continuously supply your body with high quality fuel in the form of fresh, natural and whole foods that will provide your body with all the essential nutrients to ensure everything is running smoothly. You need all the energy to power you through the most intense workout of your life.

Stay away from all processed junk that is so high in calories with very little nutritional value which will only serve to slow down your weight loss goals.

Hydration is also very important because it helps replenish all the water you lose when sweating. Water also helps improve your metabolism so when combined with tabata, it is a double threat and you achieve your weight loss goals faster.

Although you can incorporate tabata into virtually all exercise regimens, the choice of exercise you make can help you lose weight faster. The best choices are those that work on a large number of muscle groups. It is important to note that it is very normal to experience soreness for the first week of your HIIT Tabata training. But, your body will slowly adjust and you will only feel slightly sore after more training.

Here is a list of some of the most effective exercises when incorporated with tabata:

- Bicep curls
- Mountain climber
- Flys
- Burpees
- Squats
- Sit ups
- Sprints
- Bench press
- Pull ups
- Deadlifts
- Tricep dips

- Crunches
- Stairs
- Calf raises
- Leg raises
- Shoulder press

Whatever exercise you chose to incorporate with tabata training, it will raise your heart rate and metabolism almost instantly. The fact that you are performing these exercises at a high pace and intensity, your body will be forced to work harder than usual to keep up. This will propel your heart rate as it works harder to pump blood faster to all your organs and your metabolism too will be forced to jump; a very good thing especially when you are trying to shed body fat.

The amazing thing is that your metabolism will not just stay high during the workout but up to 24 hours after your workout as we had seen earlier. This simply means that your body will be torching away the fat even when lying down after your tabata training.

I can't emphasize more on the fact that virtually all exercises can incorporate tabata training for maximum weight loss benefits. We are now going to look at a very effective sample tabata routine that you can do right from home.

Tabata Exercise Regimen Example:

- Push ups
- Medicine ball lams
- Squats
- Jumping rope

Directions:

- Start with 20 seconds of power pushups (dong as many reps as you possibly can), take a 10 seconds rest.
- Next do 20 seconds of medicine all slams and rest for 10 seconds
- Do squats for 20 seconds and again rest for 10seconds.
- Lastly, skip as fast as you can for 20 seconds then rest for 10 seconds.

To make this tabata routine even more badass, repeat these sets eight more times bringing this to a total of sixteen minutes.

Once you are more comfortable and get the hang of things, you can create as many as three tabata routines, introducing a new set of exercises in every routine you do. This will keep your muscles guessing and your body will always respond anew to the challenge at hand and so you can be sure of maximum fat burn in each session.

Important!!!

Doing dynamic stretches is the best way to prepare your body for the oncoming rigorous exercises. Forget about bending down to touch your toes, ride a stationary bike for 5 minutes on low or do a steady jog for 5minutes. This will warm up your body in readiness for an intense workout.

Tabata will help increase your endurance threshold and the best part is that you will be burning all the unwanted fat way after your workout!

Pyramid exercises are great for an intense workout and ultimate burnout. A typical HIIT pyramid consists of five rounds. Increase your reps by five for the first three rounds and decrease the reps by five for the last two rounds. For example;

- Set 1 – 10 reps
- Set 2 – 15 reps
- Set 3 – 20 reps
- Set4 – 15 reps
- Set 5 – 10 reps

Pyramids can be applied to virtually all exercises, but when starting but, you can apply it on the following;

- Reverse push ups
- Lunges
- Burpees and
- Squats
- Super killer HII Set

When in the mood to take your body to the extreme limit, you can apply the above pyramid set for the following exercises for the most powerful workout session

- L Sits – put your body on a hanging position and keep your legs parallel to the ground as you pull your body as high up as possible and hold for 20 seconds.
- Ninja jumps – start from a kneeing position then jump up straight to a squat position.
- Row and clean
- Burpees

These workouts will power you through the week and help you lose weight faster than you had envisioned.

Conclusion

There is one very important point that I would like
you to remember all through your fitness life there is
no single one size fits all approach when it comes to
the best and most effective way to lose weight and
certainly High Intensity Interval Training. We are all
made very uniquely. There are some of us who only
need to do a few aerobic exercises and the fat starts
melting away while there are some of us who have to
incorporate weight exercises into HIIT workouts for
good weight loss results.

The important thing is to learn to listen to your body.
By now, you know how your body responds to certain
foods and to exercise routines. Stick to these that your
body thrives in ensuring that you are constantly
switching up things so your body doesn't end up
getting complacent.

Some of us could have reservations about performing
HIIT exercises as they seem to really be hard on your
body. However, the thing is, your body is much
stronger than you could be giving it credit for. It
doesn't matter whether you are suffering from chronic

illness, HIIT exercises will change your health and attitude towards life for the best.

In actual fact, numerous studies have shown that regular HIIT exercises reduce symptoms of and protect from chronic illnesses such as Parkinson's disease, Alzheimer's, Cancers, Stroke and so on. This has been attributed to the fact that circulation is made more efficient and also to the fact that hormonal balance is restored in individuals who regularly perform HIIT exercises.

Aside from physical health benefits, you are going to get added benefits such as a better sleep pattern, you will be a bouncing ball of energy, you are going to be a generally happier person and won't have to worry about depression, you are going to achieve your weight loss goals making you very happy and satisfied person and thus all sectors of your life are going to benefit.

There is really no reason stopping you from being a HIIT bunny. You can complain that you don't have time to exercise because at the very least, all you need is four minutes. You also can't say that gym enrollment is expensive or that you can't squeeze in time to go to the gm; you can do most HIIT exercises from the comfort of your own living room.

The most important thing really is to clearly define your goals, teach yourself how to perform HIIT exercises so your body starts getting used to activity and slowly but surely get into intensive routines that are going to see you lose weight and become a very healthy and happy person.

Life is a matter of a series of very important choices. Your health should always come at the top of the list and this involves a solid fitness regimen and a healthy and natural diet, not forgetting better sleep as this is when your body fully recovers from the strenuous HIIT workouts. With this three, your life is going to be easy breezy and weight problems will be a very distant memory!

I want you to thank yourself for wanting to change and I hope you walk away inspired or smarter.

As you read on you will find tips used by entrepreneurs, and motivational thoughts that come from coaches and entrepreneurs themselves. Have Fun and good luck with your endeavors. Before moving on, I just want to remind you that we are all born on this earth as equals. Some may have more support than others, but we can only characterize ourselves by our own actions. In other words, everyone in this world has potential hidden in a box. Some choose to find a way to open it, and some just leave it there.

Think about this and try to figure out who you are.

Some may be okay living an average life, but then there are also others who constantly look for better.

Life Hacking Tips Used by the Entrepreneurs!
Coffee Nap

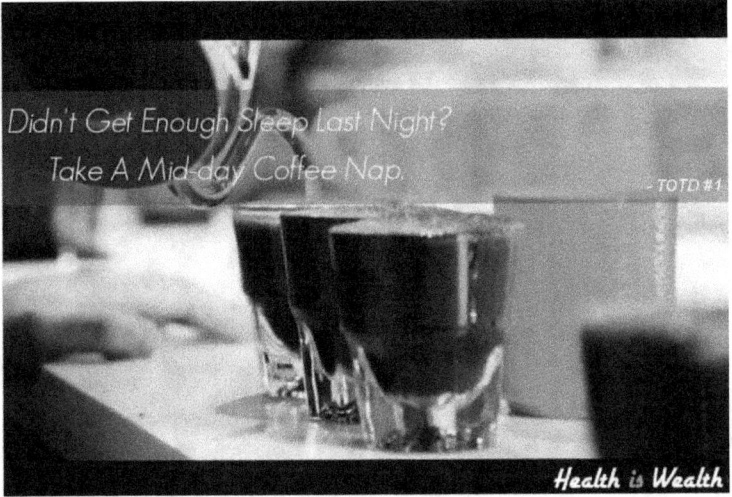

This method provided is called, "Caffeine Nap", where you drink a cup of coffee and nap for 15 minutes. The 15 minutes gives you time to rest and allows the caffeine to travel through your gastro-intestinal tract. This will provide you with a refreshing reboot by the time you wake up. But don't go over the 15-20 minutes limit or else you'll wake up in a sleepy state.

Plan the Night Before

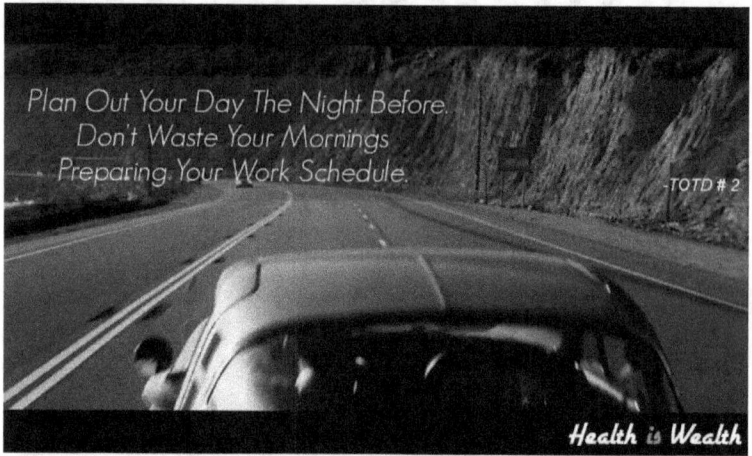

You heard of this before, you can either work hard or work smart. It's your choice. There's nothing wrong about working hard, but what's the point of working hard if the results are not there. You need to work smart and change up your routine so that your work is actually effective. Tonight before you go to bed, plan out your work for the next day so that you don't waste time in the morning. Don't waste your mornings on planning out what you want to work on as you are wasting your brains fuel. Your brain is packed with fuel from last night's rest, so go use it on something productive. Don't be like the majority of people who sit on their desk wondering what they need to do. Hope this helps!

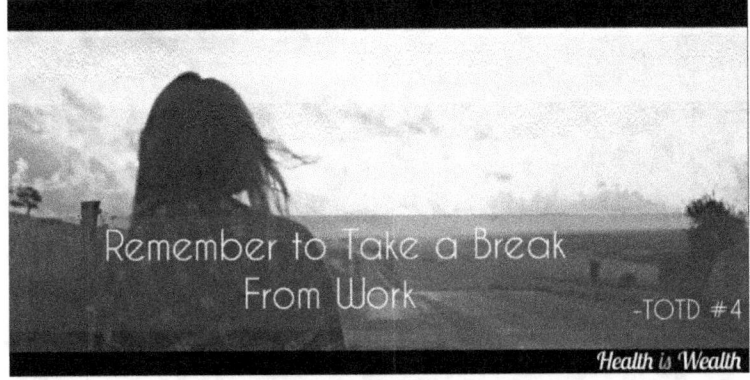

Remember to Take a Break
From Work

-TOTD #4

Health is Wealth

Most of us work for a living, and sometimes we work so hard that we feel too tired to spend time with the people we love. Just remember that our work will always change, but our family will always be there. On another thought, we need to take breaks during excessive periods of work, so that we can replenish our thoughts. Take a walk and get some fresh air.

Motivation for Those Who Want to Succeed
Are You Committed?

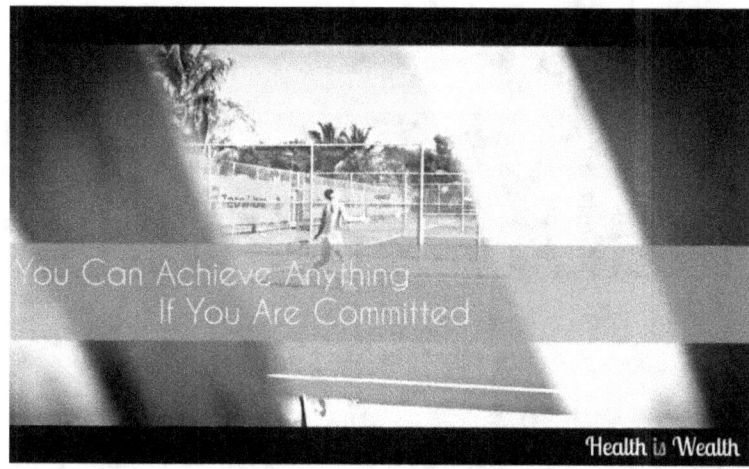

Are you interested or are you committed to achieving your current goals? Most may ask, what is the difference? If you have interest in fulfilling your goals, then you will complete your task and never look back. In other words, you will do things the same way as how most people do it. However, if you are committed to your situation, then you will find yourself working more than you need to, and trying to improve your current goals, although they are already good enough. Successful entrepreneurs are successful because they have a purpose behind their tasks, it is more than just interest. So just ask yourself, are you interested or are you committed to what you are currently doing.

There Should Never Be a Plan "B"

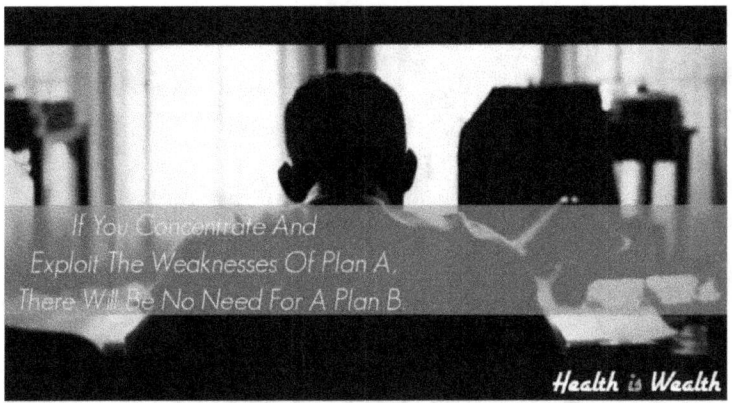

You've all heard of Plan B's. They are there to back you up just in case Plan A doesn't work. But what's the point of spending half your time on Plan A and half your time on Plan B. Instead, use your time to focus solely on Plan A so that you can perfect it. A perfect plan is better than two average plans. I've always grown up being told "If you do it right the first time, you won't have to do it a second time". So why do it a second time, you're just wasting energy. Perfect your 1st attempt so that you can move on and accomplish other things in life.

Become a Warrior

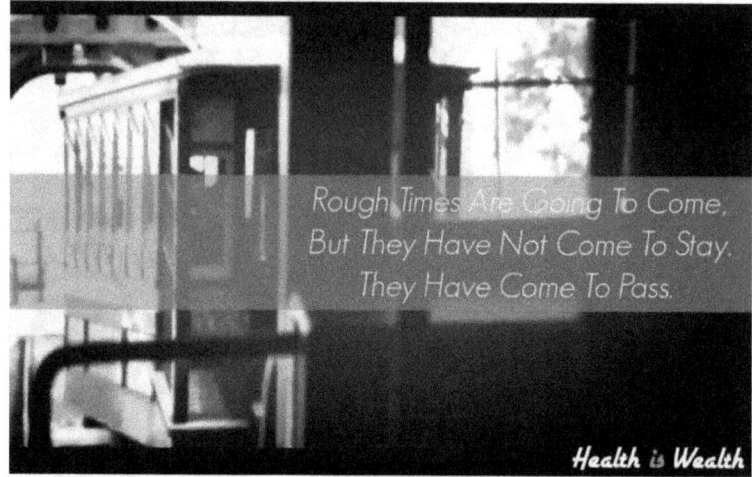

Rough Times Are Going To Come,
But They Have Not Come To Stay.
They Have Come To Pass.

Health is Wealth

It's not like we're never going to get hurt in life. And it's not like these episodes are meant to devastate us. These harsh times are just the flow of life and everyone gets them, we just need to do our part and accept them. It may sound easy but it really isn't. To accept tragedy or a mishap in your life is going to be hard because we're humans. We're emotional and that's understandable, but what about life. Life isn't going to wait for you, it's like a train with no brakes. The Sun is still going to shine, and the Moon is still going to glow. So try not to mourn for too long. These hard times are bound to come, but they have not come to stay. They have come to pass.

A Forgotten Lifestyle

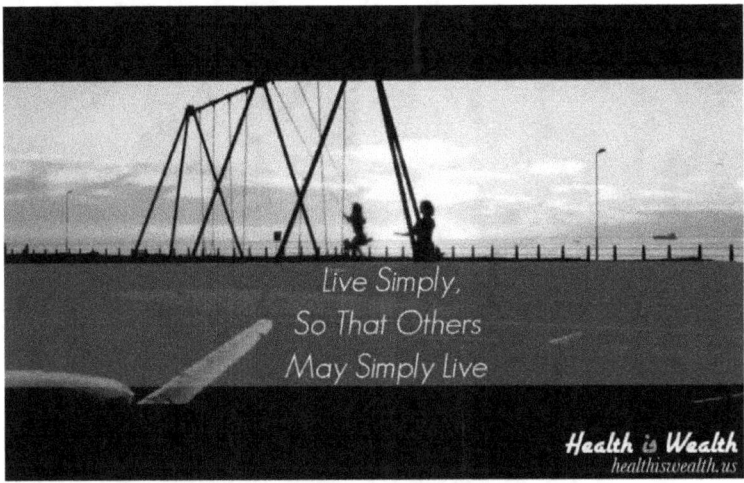

This is probably going to be my favorite for a while. Live simply, so that others may simply live. A simple saying that would do wonders for the world. In a world where capitalism is King, we often get carried away by lavish lifestyles that we envy of others. There's nothing wrong with treating yourself after a hard day's work. It's just that sometimes we become a bit too selfish. There are many people around us that aren't even able to even eat 3 times a day, and here we are complaining about getting the newest gadgets. Our job to live simply is not going to kill us. We may miss out on getting a few designer handbags or suits, but at the end of the day those funds will allow the unfortunate to live another day.

Stop Waiting and Just Do It

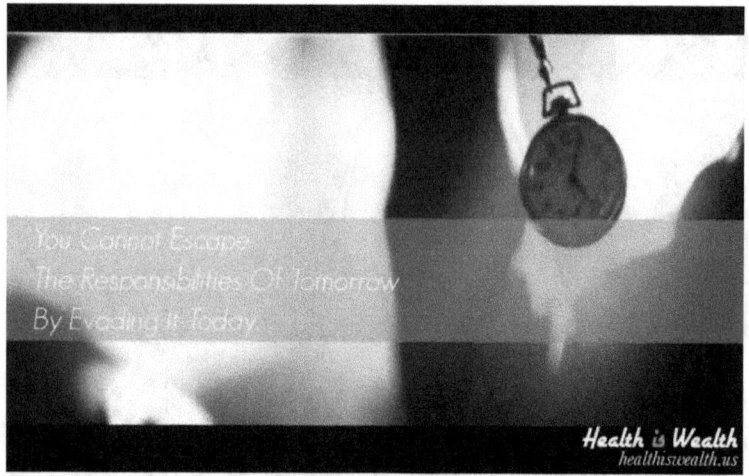

I'll do it later. For some reason we only feel obliged to start working when the deadline is near. Maybe you just need pressure to start working. We all put off work until later and our work becomes faulty when we're done. No time left to correct your mistakes. But that's not how successful people succeed and we need to instill in our minds to organize your workload so that you don't do last minute work.

You Are Only One Person, But...

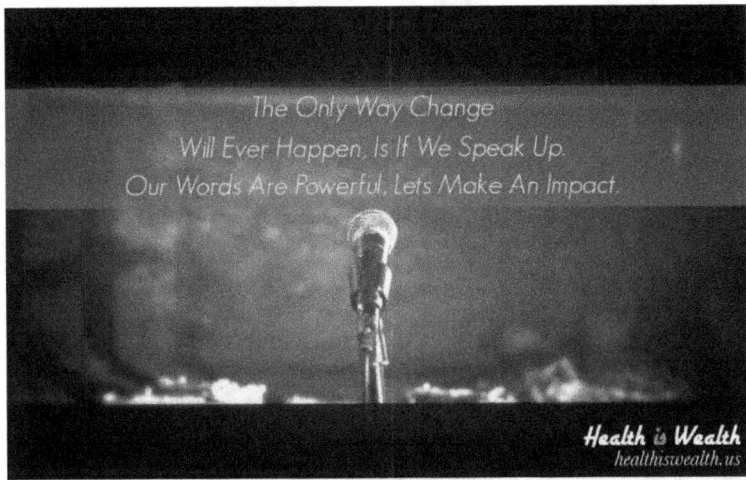

The Only Way Change
Will Ever Happen, Is If We Speak Up.
Our Words Are Powerful, Lets Make An Impact.

Health is Wealth
healthiswealth.us

This was always my problem. I'm guilty of the, "but I'm just one person" crime. I'm so used to assuming that other people are going to make an effort to change their surroundings that I suppose my input wouldn't make a difference. So what if you're just one person. If you're making a change and people around you see it, then they'll be inspired to make the change with you. You are never just one. There may be many others in the room who have the same idea as you, but are not confident enough to share. Stand up and speak your mind so that confidence may grow in them too. The only way change will ever happen, is if we speak up. Our words are powerful, let's make an impact. Don't ever think of yourself as just one.

My Dream Never Faded. Your Doubts Just made it More Clear to Me

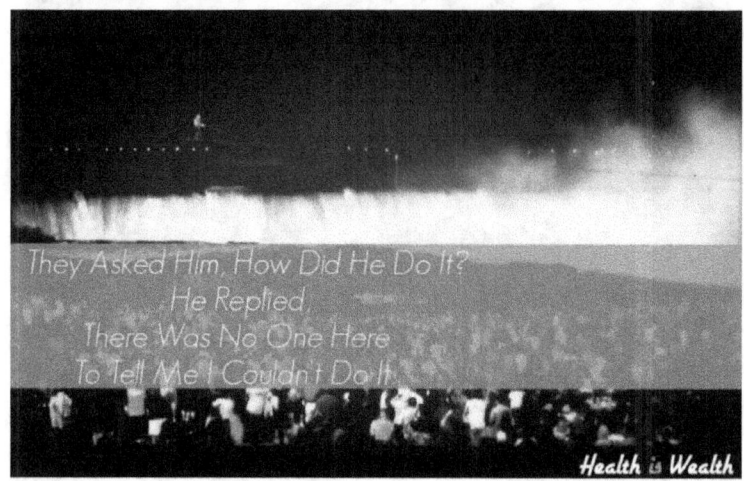

They Asked Him, How Did He Do It?
He Replied,
There Was No One Here
To Tell Me I Couldn't Do It

Health is Wealth

Are you sure? No one has ever done it before, so how will you do it? It's Impossible.

Well that's not new. People telling you what's possible and what's impossible. But what do they know. They don't know how much time and effort you put in every day and night into your work. If they tell you that it's impossible, let it fuel your fire. Proving people wrong was always a hobby of mine. So go out there and work. And when that day comes, you could tell your doubters that it was always possible.

Even if no one sees it for you, you must see it for yourself. And just like that you are on the road to success.

How's Your Willpower?

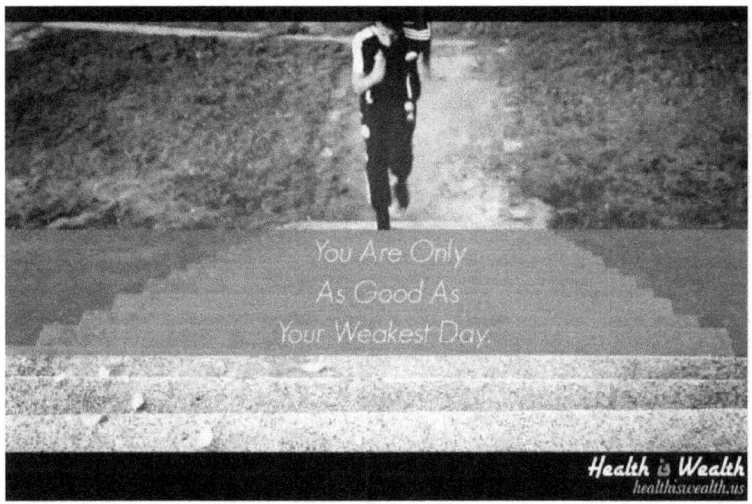

Stop setting goals and stopping half way. Sometimes we get inspired and decide to dream big. And after the next day the inspiration is gone and we decide to quit. The problem is not that we have set your goals too high. There's no such thing as setting your goals too high. The problem is us. If we don't want it bad enough, then we will be like the majority of people who start something and then say it's getting nowhere. Well don't expect results to come in just a couple of days, this is a long term commitment. We have to be committed to what we do in order to get far. We can start and end half way, but what does that really say about our willpower. You are only as good as your weakest day.

We Used to Dream a Lot

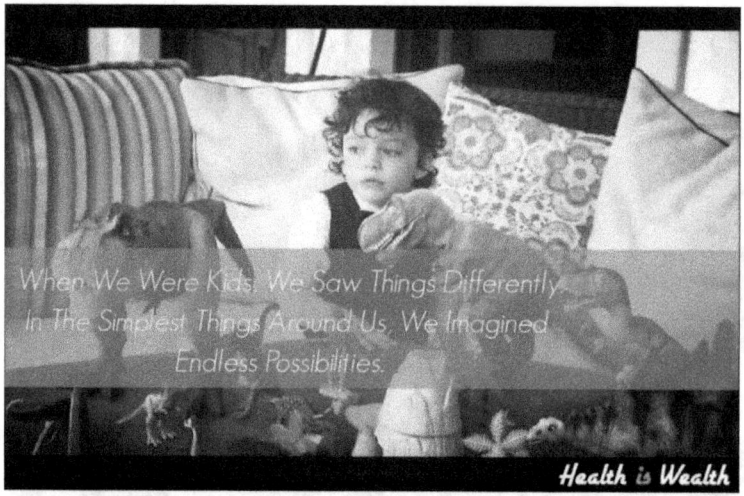

When We Were Kids, We Saw Things Differently.
In The Simplest Things Around Us, We Imagined
Endless Possibilities.

Health is Wealth

Back then we used to tie a towel around our neck and jump off our beds only to soar for a couple of seconds. But those couple of seconds were enough to allow us to feel like superheroes. We turned that towel into a cape and it gave us an identity. When we were kids, we saw things differently. In the simplest things around us, we imagined endless possibilities. Who would have known that a chunk of metal would help us fly around the world? That's absurd right? It's hard to imagine an airplane from looking at a chunk of metal. As we grow older we slowly push our imaginations aside, and that towel that used to help us fly is just a rag to us now. We've grown up in a world filled with pessimists, whom only know how to provide doubts into our imaginations. It's hard to be innovative when we have so much doubts in our own ideas. So just let those imaginations come back and give them another chance. You'll never know where those imaginations will take you.

G.R.I.N.D.

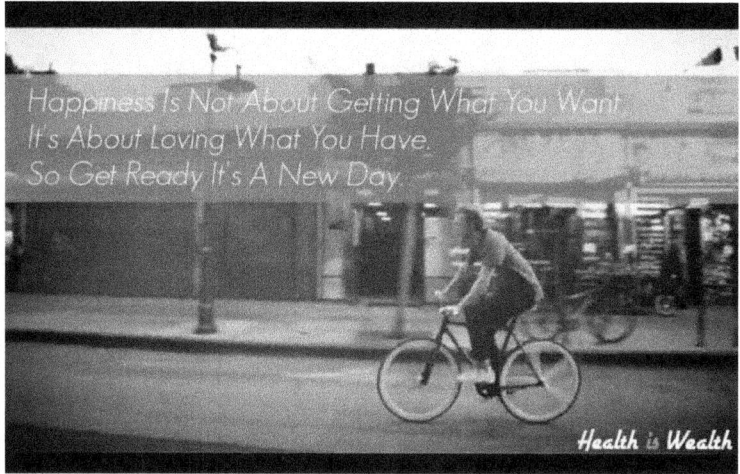

Sometimes I feel like I'm not making any progress toward my goals and it frightens me. My dreams and goals are still there, but I have my doubts like any human would. So today I turned on my speakers and Asher Roth was on. It was only then that I realized that I was doing it all wrong. My goal was to work hard so that I could buy my parents stuff that they would be happy to have. I wanted them to be happy. I wanted them to know that in the near future, their working hours would be lessened and that I would bombard them with gifts.

But it wasn't until today, that I realize how faulty my goals were. I was so focused on spending time on work for a better future that I nearly forgot about spending time with my parents in the present. Spending money on my parents can come a little later, but for now it's about spending time with the people you love. Happiness isn't not about getting what you want all the time, it's about loving what you have. So get ready, it's a new day.

Appreciate What You Have!

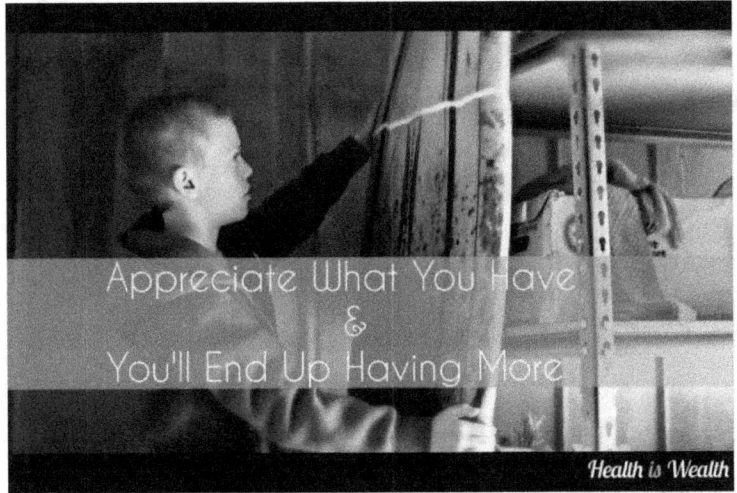

Today we are so focused with getting new things that we neglect what we already have. We look forward to creating new relationships, and leave behind the relationships we already have. Instead of trying to fix the problems in our current situations, we look for something new as a solution, but at the end of the day we are just dragging out the problem. So let's fix something today, before looking elsewhere. When a friendship is confronted with problems, they settle the problem with each other and grow stronger together.

Stuck in Your Comfort Zone?

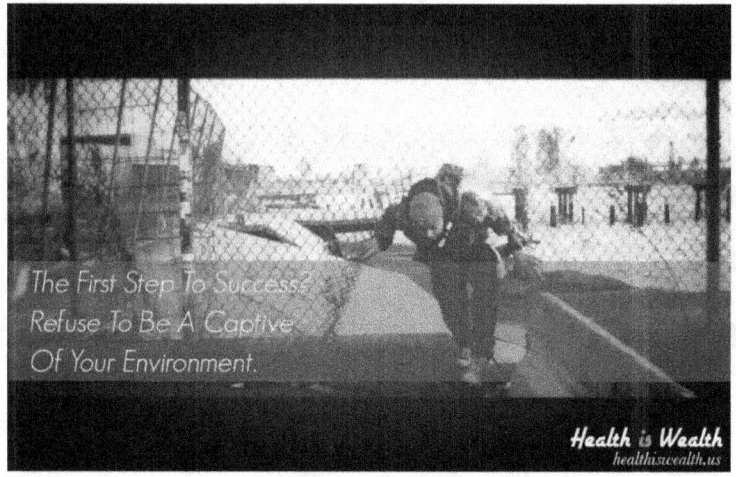

The First Step To Success?
Refuse To Be A Captive
Of Your Environment.

Health is Wealth
healthiswealth.us

You say you want to be healthy. You say you want to be rich. But are you doing anything towards these goals. Surrounding yourself with a room full of junk food is not going to help. Neither is hanging around people who don't believe in working hard. You need to get out of your old environment and go find a new one. Stop being trapped in the misery that is around you. Go meet new friends that actually care about the wellness of their body and people who set new goals every week. Once you are in their environment, you'll find yourself trying to work as hard as or even harder than them. Place yourself in a healthy environment, but first you have to leave your old one.

Thank you for taking the time to read this book and may you always have a perfectly balanced life. If you haven't already read my author's description before purchasing this book, you would know that I am also the founder of Finicky. The images provided by the book come from my website, "Finicky.us"

Preview of "Public Speaking: 7 Essentials Steps Used by Top Entrepreneurs"
You may purchase this book by <u>clicking here</u>

Or by using this link <u>http://amzn.to/1dsxVg9</u>

The feeling of nervousness or stage-fright when presenting to an audience is perfectly normal. Even the best public speakers still get nervous. This is a part of being human, we are wired to be worried about our reputation and public speaking is a threat to us. In psychological terms, our fight or flight responses comes into play and our body starts feeling different.

Before I go on any further, I would just like to tell you that the fears of public speaking are not to be overcome, we need to adapt to our public speaking environment. I would like you to keep this in mind as you continue to read on.

Before considering talking in public there are some things you must be aware of. The first thing you should do before speaking in public is to find out who you are and what you need.

The feedback you will receive after speaking in public is relevant for what you are going to do next. You should always meditate and answer these questions: Who am I? What do I want? What do I need?